Healthy Gut, Healthy Mind, Healthy Life…

A Healthy Approach To the Microbiome

Best Life Publishing L.L.C

For permission requests, please get in touch with the publisher at the email address below:

Elizabeth Ann Watt

Liz@ElizabethAnnWatt.com

ISSN: 978-1-963234-01-5

"All disease begins in the gut."
—Hippocrates

INDEX

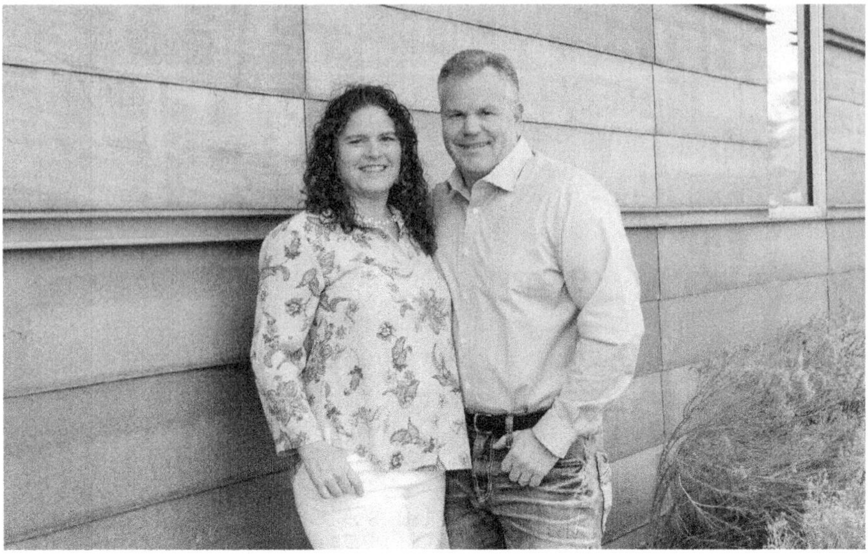

ABOUT THE AUTHORS

Dr. M. Shane and Elizabeth Watt, known as Shane and Liz by many, have been married for over 30 years and are parents to 6 children. They live in the Salt Lake Valley and are committed to helping others regain their health. They have created a business called Elevated Learning, where they stand by their motto of Give Knowledge, Empower Others, and Elevate Lives. They work in the same office, seeing each other's patients and clients. They are speakers and educators in their field.

Together, they put on the largest natural health conference in the West, the Be Healthy Utah Natural Health and Wellness

Conference. They have created a platform where others can learn about natural health through education, products, and services. They are looking to expand their conference soon to other states in the West.

Dr.Shane Watt

Dr. Watt owns and is the clinical director of Mountain West Chiropractic and Neurobolic Health Center.

Dr. Watt is a Chiropractic Physician located in South Jordan, Utah. He graduated from Life Chiropractic College West in 1996 with clinical honors.

Dr. Watt always strives to give his patients the best treatment possible. It is essential for him to continue his education in the field to stay on top of his game. Keeping up with the latest research is his top priority. He is on a board that associates with a group of highly educated Doctors around the country, creating, inventing, and implementing new cutting-edge treatments to help their patients.

Dr. Watt not only provides chiropractic care but also specializes in functional health. Functional Health looks at the underlying factors of health problems and why the patient is experiencing these symptoms. After being in practice for 13 years doing strict chiropractic care, he began evolving his practice into helping those suffering from chronic health conditions. Many were hopeless because they could not find any help in the standard medical model. This did not sit well with Dr. Watt, so he began his quest to find answers for these patients. Through his implementation of holistic treatments, many patients now had answers and were able to regain their new health journey.

Liz Watt

Liz Watt is a public speaker, author, and Holistic Wellness Expert. She educates others on how the mind, body, and soul harmonize. Each part of our bodies is emotionally, physically, or spiritually interconnected. She founded Journey of Healing, a mentorship program combining these three life aspects. Her online programs emphasize that all three areas must be balanced for proper healing.

Liz has experienced many health Challenges throughout her adult life. Through her natural healing process, she has become an expert in holistic health. Liz is passionate about educating others on the importance of giving our bodies what they need to heal.

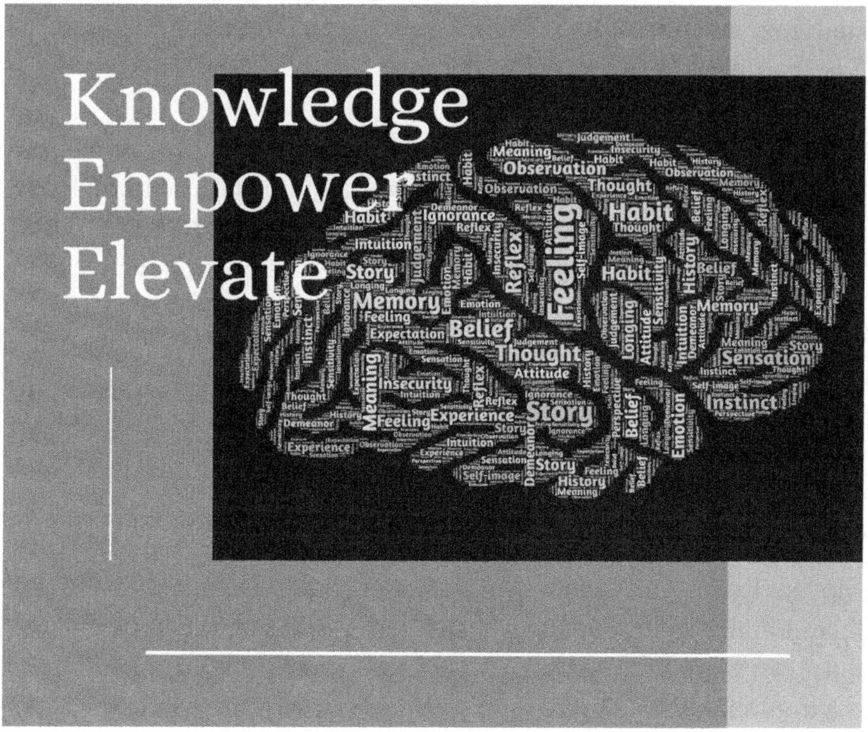

Chapter One

Give Knowledge, Empower Others, Elevate Lives
Give Knowledge

One of the most important things we can do is acquire knowledge. We are creatures of habit. Our brains are wired to learn, ponder, and act on that knowledge. One principle we stand on is always to give knowledge to others. We feel it is our responsibility to pass this knowledge on to you. We are educators first. Because of the knowledge we have acquired through countless hours of reading, studying, and attending seminars, we can help many individuals live their best, healthiest lives.

Empower Others

We become more empowered when we acquire and use knowledge in our lives. The more knowledge we have, the more we can improve our lives and the lives around us. We both believe we are all capable of being in control of our health. We empower others by giving them the knowledge to improve themselves constantly. As we each focus on our health, we become empowered with tools to help aid our bodies in healing.

Elevate Lives

Our main goal while working with our clients and patients is to Elevate Lives. Only when we give others knowledge and empower them to take control of their health can we elevate the lives of those we work with. By arming ourselves and creating a healing environment, we can live more meaningful, productive, and healthy lives.

We have created this book to provide you with extensive knowledge in a simple, easy-to-understand format. This will equip you with the tools to feel empowered and make the necessary changes. As you begin your healing journey, know matter where you started, your life will be elevated.

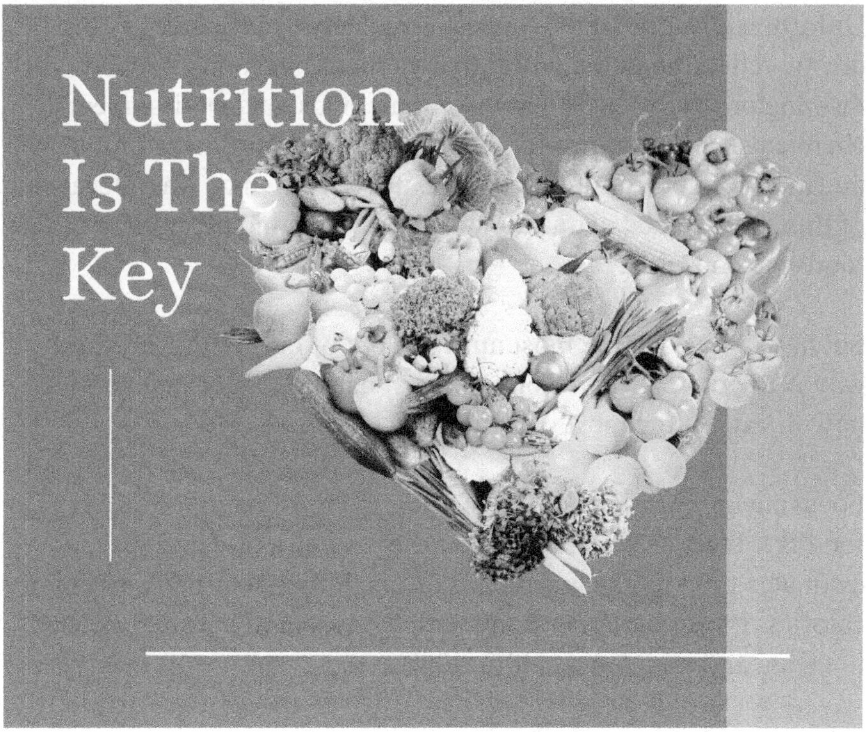

Chapter Two

It All Begins with Nutrition

Our bodies run on nutrition. Vitamins, minerals, and water fuel our cells to create life within us. Without these vitamins, minerals, and water, our bodies' cells begin to die off and do not create an environment for healing. Our goal in healing our bodies is to create a healing environment. Our bodies are brilliant, and they know what they need to survive.

Unfortunately, one of the biggest obstacles we face today is the drastic reduction in the nutritional value of our foods. Modern farming practices, livestock-raising methods, and environmental chemicals have significantly depleted the nutrients in our food. The nutrition we get from food today is not what it once was. Because of this, we must be extra cautious when selecting the quality of the foods we consume.

So, how do we get the most nutrition out of our foods? The best way is to get your food from the most natural source and know how to extract the most nutrition.

Focusing on nutrition and consuming the most natural form of your food is known as a nutrient-dense diet. A nutrient-dense diet evaluates food by the nutrition it offers to fuel your body, not by its calories. It provides your body with the essential nutrients needed to create and maintain healthy cells.

Like we said, our bodies are competent and know what we need. Our job is to give our bodies what they need so they can do their job in return.

No wonder disease is so prevalent right now. Our foods are depleted in nutrition, and our bodies are not given the proper tools to produce healthy and vibrant cells. Because of this, our bodies cannot work at their peak performance. Giving our bodies what they need could eradicate many sicknesses and diseases.

Because our foods are so depleted in nutrition, the effects of the chemicals, pesticides, and herbicides in our environment, and the gross negligence of antibiotic use in the meat industry, inflammation within our bodies is on the rise. Inflammation is directly correlated to all chronic health conditions.

How do we know this? Dr. Watt has worked with many patients who have had a variety of illnesses that have affected their lives. By changing their diets and reducing inflammation, their bodies have healed, and they no longer suffer from diseases like they once did.

Liz's Own Health Battle

I was one of those patients who suffered greatly. Over the last 20 years, my life declined to a point where it was hard to function and overcome illness. My body was in a constant cycle of pain and inflammation. It wasn't until I addressed the inflammation nutritionally that my symptoms started to disappear.

So, what were these changes? One of the first things I started to notice was I no longer had constipation, which I had dealt with for decades. The PH problem I had for five years vanished. I no longer had continual burning in my sensitive areas. I could use soap in the shower, and intimacy would no longer hurt. After a couple of months, my corn sensitivity was under control. My eyesight even improved, and I no longer needed to wear glasses. I had a prior sensitivity to metals and could finally wear earrings. My body was numb, and my skin no longer felt any sensations. By incorporating proper nutrition, this was drastically improved. My energy increased, and my mood was happier. But the biggest thing I noticed that trumped everything: I was out of constant pain and was finally "LIVING."

I also saw miracles in my family and others. My daughter's eczema went away, my son's allergies disappeared, and many people who I worked with also had similar results with much more healing. Talk about miracles!

Realizing I needed to do more to improve my health, I began to decrease my sugar levels, consume little gluten, concentrate on minerals, increase gut-healing foods, and cook and focus on nutrient-dense foods. With these changes, the numbness in my back started to heal. I had fewer painful body flare-ups, dramatically increasing my overall health.

Because of the successes of my family, clients, and Dr. Watt's patients, we felt obligated to share these important and sometimes lost truths with the world. After many long hours, we have become experts in our field.

This is why we are so passionate about what we do. We have seen and also experienced miracles by creating a healing environment. Our bodies know how to heal if we give them what they need. So, take this knowledge we are about to share with you and incorporate it into your life. Empower your own body to do what it does best. As you do this, your life will elevate, and your vitality will increase.

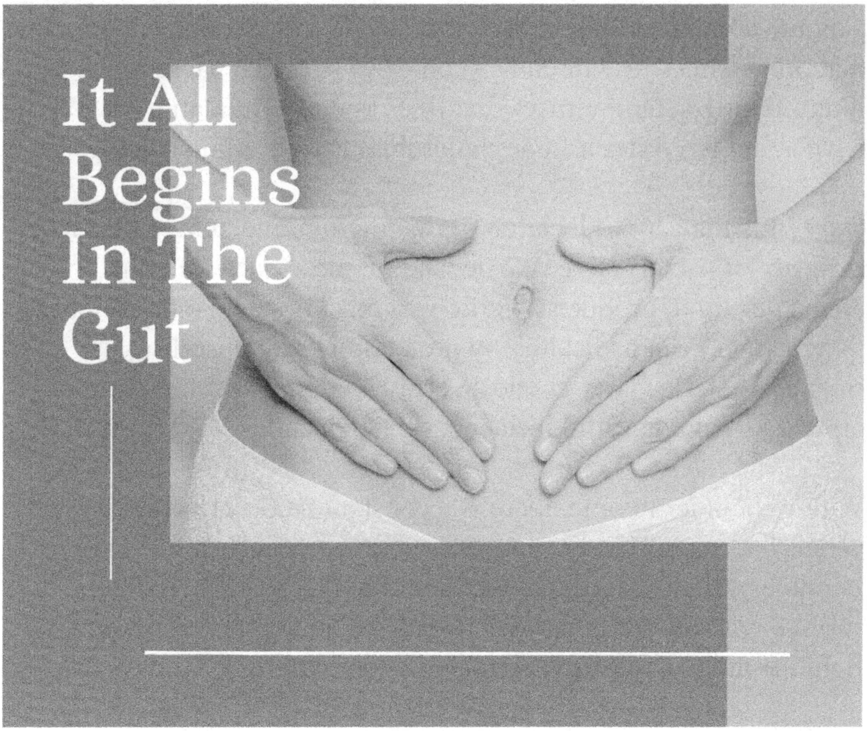

Chapter Three

Good Bugs Bad Bugs

Our bodies have trillions of bugs within them, keeping us safe and protected. The gut is the central location for these bugs, which is called the microbiome.

The microbiome is defined as the collective genomes of the microbes. A genome is an organism's complete set of DNA. Each genome contains all the information needed to build and maintain that organism. These microbes comprise bacteria, bacteriophage, fungi, protozoa, and viruses that live inside the human body. We have about ten times as many microbial cells as human cells.

Our gut is the central location of the microbiome, where the large majority of bacteria live. We depend on these bacteria to help digest our food, produce specific vitamins, regulate our immune system, and keep us healthy by protecting us against disease-causing bacteria. They create an army charging at full force to protect us from harmful influences from outside.

Within the microbiome, there is a constant battle of good bugs versus bad bugs. The bad bugs are also critical. They keep our immune system working at its optimum. Our bodies could not survive without these harmful bugs. The good bugs constantly fight off the bad bugs to keep them under control.

Unfortunately, the good bugs deteriorate and die without the right environment. If there is not an environment where the good bugs can not grow and multiply, it opens the door for the bad bugs to multiply. When the bad bugs start to multiply, unhealthy cells can also multiply. When this gets out of control, a disease can form.

Our first thought is to get rid of all bad bugs. However, getting rid of all bad bugs will do the opposite and cause your body to get sick. These bad bugs are just as critical as the good bugs. Our bodies are designed to regulate the good bug-bad bug ratio.

The best way to keep the ratio at its optimum is to feed your microbiome what it needs to stay healthy and vibrant. There are many ways to keep your microbiome healthy. You can do this by hydrating these good microbes by drinking plenty of water, eating plant-based foods, and feeding them full of healthy bugs, often known as probiotics. Just as important as probiotics are prebiotics.

A prebiotic is a non-digestible fibrous food that feeds and promotes beneficial microbes. Fine-tuning this balance is essential for your health.

Recently, we have realized the importance of probiotics and how they can benefit our microbiome. There are many ways to feed your body with probiotics. Below are some of the most common ways to achieve this.

Probiotics

Close to 1000 different strains of bacteria are present in our microbiome. Nutritional microbiologists study the best probiotic strains and how to create the best microbiome. This lets you target and fine-tune the best strain for your needs.
The most common strains of probiotics found that give you the best benefit for your microbiome are:

1. **Streptococcus thermophilus**: promotes healthy tissue in the small intestine. It discourages nitrates, like those in spinach, celery, and cured meats, from turning into harmful nitrates. It also breaks down casein, a protein in cheeses known to cause allergies.

2. **Bacillus Laterosporus:** A hearty strain that fights many harmful organisms, including candida.

3. **Pediococcus Acidilactici:** Undigested food can rot in your gut. Pediococcus Acidilactici helps prevent this. One study found that it also helps prevent harmful organisms from damaging the gut environment.

4. **Bifidobacterium Breve:** Essential for colon health, especially if

you've taken antibiotics. Studies have found that many digestive problems coincide with low levels of Bifidobacterium breve.

5. Bifidobacterium Infantis: Supports the digestive system by releasing an acid that keeps harmful organisms from taking hold. It's beneficial for people suffering from digestive ailments or occasional constipation.

6. Bifidobacterium Bifidum: A household name in probiotic strains. It keeps unwanted bacteria out, eases digestion, and boosts the immune system. It plays a vital role in immune function and allergy response. Encourages normal, healthy-looking skin.

7. Bifidobacterium Lactis: Neutralizes gluten, the wheat protein responsible for gluten sensitivity. Gluten is the culprit for many underlying sensitivities since it damages the intestinal lining and can cause a leaky gut.

8. Bifidobacterium Longum: Helps keep acid levels balanced. It's beneficial for anyone taking antibiotics.

9. Lactobacillus acidophilus: Supports digestion, particularly lactose digestion, and boosts the immune system.

10. Lactobacillus brevis: Helping out on both ends, soothing oral and colon tissue.

11. Lactobacillus Bulgaricus: Creates natural antibiotics in your gut that fight invading organisms. It also releases acids that neutralize toxins and promote balance.

12. Lactobacillus Casei: Supports digestion and the immune system and soothes the bowels.

13. Lactobacillus Gasseri: Supports digestion, balances blood sugar, and encourages an average body weight.

14. Lactococcus Lactis: Helps digestion and encourages a typical gut environment. Defend against leaky gut.

15. Lactobacillus Plantarum: The best part of this bacteria is that it produces antibiotics that intelligently target bad bacteria. This probiotic also makes lysine, an essential amino acid that supports calcium absorption and hormone production and boosts the immune system. It can live in your gut and keep pathogenic disease-causing microorganisms from flourishing. It creates a healthy barrier in your colon to keep dangerous bacteria from penetrating the lining of your intestines and entering your bloodstream.

16. Lactobacillus Paracasei: This bacteria helps with fatigue and protects teeth from cavities, and many people also report it lessens the impact of environmental sensitivities.

17. Lactobacillus rhamnosus: is generally cited for promoting a happy and healthy gut environment. It also has a reputation for helping with UTIs by kick-starting antibodies and boosting the immune system.

18. Lactobacillus salivarius: fights unwanted microbes in the mouth and small intestine. It's considered essential for oral health. Like many others, this strain thrives with prebiotic foods like bananas, barley, tomatoes, and garlic.

All of these strains are important for our microbiome. We need to cultivate our gut to create an environment where these good health-promoting strains for our gut can flourish.

Recent studies have found that targeting only a few of these strands may not be the best for your microbiome. Each bacteria needs each other to survive. Getting a wide range of beneficial bacteria will increase your odds of having a healing environment.

Unfortunately, many over-the-counter probiotics do not deliver the desired results. To be effective, probiotics must withstand the body's protective barriers.

Probiotics Downstream
1- Stomach Acid
2- Bile Salts
3- Pancreatic Enzymes
4-The Immune System
5- Being able to get along with the rest of the microflora

The sad truth is that most over-the-counter probiotics do not pass the body's natural defense mechanism and do not make it to the area in the digestive tract to be productive.

Be cautious of how probiotics are sold with more strains and millions of colonies. This is more about marketing than actual science. We have recently found the best source of probiotics to be an ancient spore form. We are now using this with our patients.

Food Source Probiotics

When pursuing a nutrient-dense diet, it is best to go to the most natural source of any nutrient. This can include vitamins and minerals, as well as probiotics and prebiotics. This is why we stress the importance of getting as many probiotics from your food source as possible.

There is considerable controversy over dairy. For those who don't struggle with dairy, there are many options you can enjoy. Plain yogurt, cottage cheese, and Kefir (fermented milk) can easily be purchased at the store for your convenience.

There are also many good alternatives for those who want to go the non-dairy route. Our favorite way to consume probiotics is through fermented vegetables, raw vinegar, and coconut kefir. Another way you can also get probiotics is in kombucha (fermented tea). We don't usually recommend this way because the sugar content can be so high that it counterbalances your microbiome. You can buy all of these in the store or make them yourself.

Miracle in a Jar

In Liz's journey, fermented vegetables were considered a "Miracle in a Jar." Fermented vegetables are easy to make, last a long time, and are filled with millions of good probiotics. When Liz started to add fermented vegetables to her diet, her health began to change drastically for the better.

Fermented vegetables are chopped-up vegetables submerged under water. Every vegetable has a bacteria called lactobacilli on its surface. Lactobacilli is a naturally occurring good bacteria. When you submerge the vegetables under water, the starches and sugars in the vegetables begin to convert to lactic acid. Lactic acid is a natural preservative that inhibits the growth of harmful bacteria.

The naturally occurring lactic acid makes the environment in the foods so acidic that the harmful bacteria cannot survive. The lactic acid keeps it at a high enough acid level that the good bacteria can survive and thrive. Through this process, a potent probiotic is formed.

The process of producing fermented vegetables is relatively easy. The required supplies are vegetables, a glass bottle, salt, and a lid. Depending on the culture you are doing, you may also want whey or starter culture.

Whey and starter culture is a way of adding good bacteria to your mix to start your process off right and give your vegetables a great starting point. This way, you can control more of the kinds of bacteria you want to produce to provide the most beneficial health results.

I prefer not to use any whey or starter culture in my batches. I enjoy the taste better without them, but it is up to you and what you prefer. You can buy starter culture on the internet.

Below is a vegetable combination we have found to be the best in taste and variety. The full recipe is in the back under “Recipes."

Start with an excellent large-size cabbage base. Your cabbage base should be around 80%, and the other items added to your mixture should only be around 20%.

-Cabbage
-Carrots
-Red Pepper
-Cilantro
-Italian Parsley
-Celery (brine)
-Sea Salt or Himalayan Salt

Salt is essential when fermenting vegetables. It creates an environment where harmful bacteria can not grow, and it also helps with the crunchiness and texture of the vegetables. There is a delicate balance when putting salt on your vegetables. Over-salting can lead to throwing out the whole batch, and under-salting can lead to mushy vegetables. A good recommendation is to salt to taste unless you are trying to preserve your vegetables for an extended time. They should taste salty but not overbearing.

Another way to increase the salt content without adding salt is to use a natural sodium base from other vegetables. We have found the best vegetable for this is celery. Juice your celery stalks and add the celery juice to your salt mixture. Stir this mixture together and add it to your vegetables. By doing this, you can cut your salt in half. Using the celery juice will keep up the sodium content, keep your vegetables crunchier, and not make your vegetables taste too salty.

To make it easy and simplify the process, Start with one head of cabbage. Remove the outer layer of your head. Cut out the center of the cabbage and set it aside. Shred the rest of the cabbage head. Shred two carrots and one red pepper. Chop the cilantro and Italian parsley and add them to the mixture. Juice one celery stalk and add one Tablespoon of Himalayan or mineralized salt. Add the salt mixture to the vegetables and set aside for 20 minutes.

After the juices have come to the surface, begin kneading your vegetables until most of the water has been extracted from your vegetables.

Place the vegetable mixture into (2) 32-oz. wide-mouth jars. Make sure to get out all the air pockets. Run a butter knife through it and push the vegetable mixture down with your fist.

Place the whole cabbage leaves over the vegetables, carefully submerging them under the brine mixture. Place the center stumps over the cabbage leaves and close your lid tight.

Because juices can escape from the bottle during fermentation, put your bottles in a deep dish and set them on your counter for 5 to 7 days. If not using a fermentation lid, It is vital to burp (quickly open) your vegetables twice daily as they accumulate gases during fermentation. Failure to do this can cause your glass jars to explode. After your fermentation time, place them in the fridge to stop the process. Your new probiotic vegetables will last in the fridge for six long months.

To get the best benefit from fermented vegetables, we have found that consuming 1-2 tablespoons twice a day is best. When starting this new protocol, it is essential to start slow. Start by having only ½ tsp twice daily and work your way up. Some people enjoy having them plain, while others like to add them to their salads or a dash of sesame oil. However, if you decide to have them, it is up to you. The most important thing is that you have them.

On rare occasions, some people may begin with mild flu-like symptoms. This is normal, and you should not be afraid. Your body is shedding away all the harmful bacteria in your gut. If you have excess gas or flu-like symptoms, cut back a little and work your way up. Eventually, your body will regulate, and you can consume them with each meal.

Below are some links to a series called "Learning with Liz." They will show you step-by-step how to make fermented vegetables, raw vinegar, and other items to help naturally heal your gut and body.

http://yourjourneyofhealing.com/learning-with-liz/
http://www.watthealth.com/learning-with-liz.php

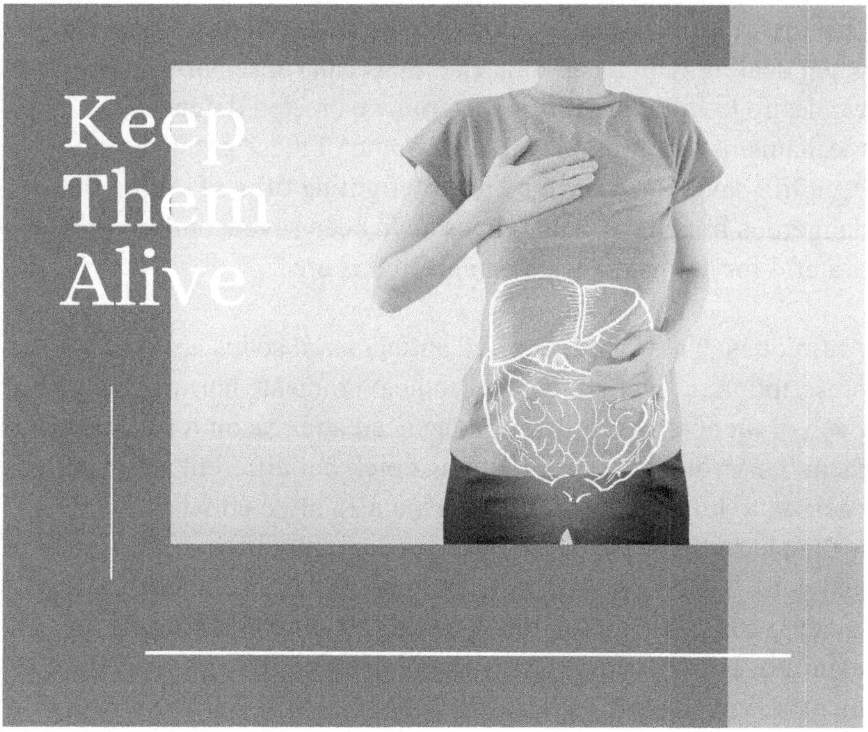

Chapter Four

Keeping Those Good Bugs Alive

We must keep all our cells healthy for our bodies to be healthy. As discussed in the previous chapter, there must be a good ratio between the good and bad bugs. The bad bugs are just as critical as the good bugs. Because of this, we must exercise extra caution to preserve both sides.

Our first reaction when we think of any bug is to kill it, especially when dealing with a bad bug. Bad bugs can cause harm. Because we desire to kill all harmful bacteria, we created defense mechanisms to aid in this process. Some of these practices have been life-saving and have helped by fighting off and killing these dangerous infections. Many lives have been saved, and we are grateful for medical advancements in this area.

Antibiotics, hand sanitizers, and antibacterial soaps are sold by prescription or over the counter to help eradicate harmful bacteria. Each of them has their own unique need and reason for having them. Unfortunately, we cannot just pick out different strains of bacteria to kill. The good bacteria are also affected when we fight off the harmful bacteria. Yes, you are lowering both the destructive and good bacteria counts. Your ratio between good and bad bacteria can often be affected, and other symptoms or diseases can manifest. Because of this, it is essential to exercise extra caution to increase your supply of healthy bacteria.

Antibiotics

Antibiotics have genuinely been lifesavers. We are very grateful for them, as they have saved many lives that would have been lost. Our biggest concern with antibiotics is their overuse. When antibiotics are overused, your body develops something called antibiotic resistance.

Antibiotic resistance is a widespread problem that the Centers for Disease Control and Prevention (CDC) calls "one of the world's most pressing public health problems." Bacteria that were once highly responsive to antibiotics have become increasingly resistant.

Pneumococcal infections (which cause pneumonia, ear infections, sinus infections, and meningitis), skin infections, and tuberculosis are becoming more challenging to treat. In addition to antibiotic resistance, overusing antibiotics can lead to other problems.

Antibiotics kill many different bacteria, even the good ones that help keep the body healthy. Sometimes, antibiotics can cause a person to develop diarrhea due to a lack of good bacteria that help digest food properly. In some cases, harmful bacteria, like Clostridium difficile, known as C diff, may overgrow and cause infections.

Antibacterial Soap

Antibacterial soap was put on the market to eradicate the bad bacteria that spread from one person to another. This is very important in certain instances, such as when a doctor is going into surgery.

Recently, the FDA warned against using antibacterial soaps and the harm they cause.

According to the U.S. Food and Drug Administration (FDA), there isn't enough science to show that over-the-counter antibacterial soaps are better at preventing illness than washing with plain soap and water. The benefits of using antibacterial hand soap haven't been proven. In addition, the wide use of these products over a long time has raised the question of potential adverse effects on your health.

Moreover, antibacterial soap products contain chemical ingredients, such as triclosan and triclocarban, which may carry unnecessary risks because their benefits are unproven. By using these types of soaps, you are exposing your family to unnecessary chemicals. Some manufacturers have begun to revise these products to remove these ingredients.

Hand Sanitizer

It wasn't that long ago when our hands got dirty; we found a sink and washed them. In the 1990s, hand sanitizer was introduced, and a sink was no longer needed. In our fast-paced society, hand sanitizer is an accessible, convenient item. Now you will find a hand.

Hand sanitizers are in every classroom, on many key chains, and in almost every bathroom. In the market, there is no end to hand sanitizer's many ways to help us stay clean and healthy.

Hand sanitizers were invented by those who work in the medical field. In the hospital, keeping hands free of bacteria and viruses is vital to avoid spreading them from patient to patient. Hand sanitizers can be handy as doctors and nurses are often rushed in their daily activities.

Hand sanitizers create dry skin. The alcohol in them removes all of the natural oils on your skin, which are your natural defense system. By eliminating these oils, you are left with dry skin and lose your most crucial barrier to your body. Hand sanitizers accelerate aging and damage your skin cells.

The fragrances in hand sanitizers can also be dangerous. Since manufacturers are not required to list fragrance ingredients on the label, you don't know what you're exposing yourself to. Many fragrances are irritating and have been linked to allergies and hormone disruption.

Glyphosate, In Other Words, Weed Killers

Glyphosate is an herbicide. It is applied to the leaves of plants to kill both broadleaf plants and grasses. The sodium salt form of glyphosate regulates plant growth and ripens fruit.

Glyphosate was first registered for use in the U.S. in 1974 and is one of the most widely used herbicides in the country.

Weeds can be so annoying. Anything to remove them would help with our gardening and flower beds. Because of this, many people flocked to buy this product.

Monsanto, the company that invented Roundup, genetically engineered seeds to grow food crops that could tolerate high doses of Roundup. With these new genetically engineered seeds, farmers could now easily control weeds on their crops. Crops thrived while Roundup wiped out the weeds around them.

Wanting to sell more of their herbicide, Monsanto also encouraged farmers to use Roundup as a desiccant to dry out all their crops so they could harvest them faster. So, Roundup is now routinely sprayed directly on a host of non-GMO crops.

There has been a whole slew of sickness that has been linked to glyphosate. This includes ADHD, Alzheimer's, birth defects, autism, cancer, celiac and gluten intolerance, kidney disease, colitis, depression, diabetes, heart disease, hypothyroidism, leaky gut, inflammatory diseases, pregnancy problems, obesity, and respiratory problems.

The bottom line is that we have no idea what these chemicals are doing to our bodies. There is still much to be discovered around this controversial topic. Any chemical can change the makeup of the microbiome. Consumers need to control what they eat, where they get it, and how they are prepared. Our bodies run on nutrition, and if the chemicals cause our bodies not to absorb these nutrients, it can lead to disease.

We must do everything possible to keep the good bugs alive within our microbiome, where most of our immune systems are stored. If it is not functioning correctly, diseases can be created. The more we die off the good bacteria, the more the harmful bacteria can flourish and take over. So, whether it is antibiotics or the chemicals sprayed on our foods, we need to be transparent and provide what is best for our bodies and our environment.

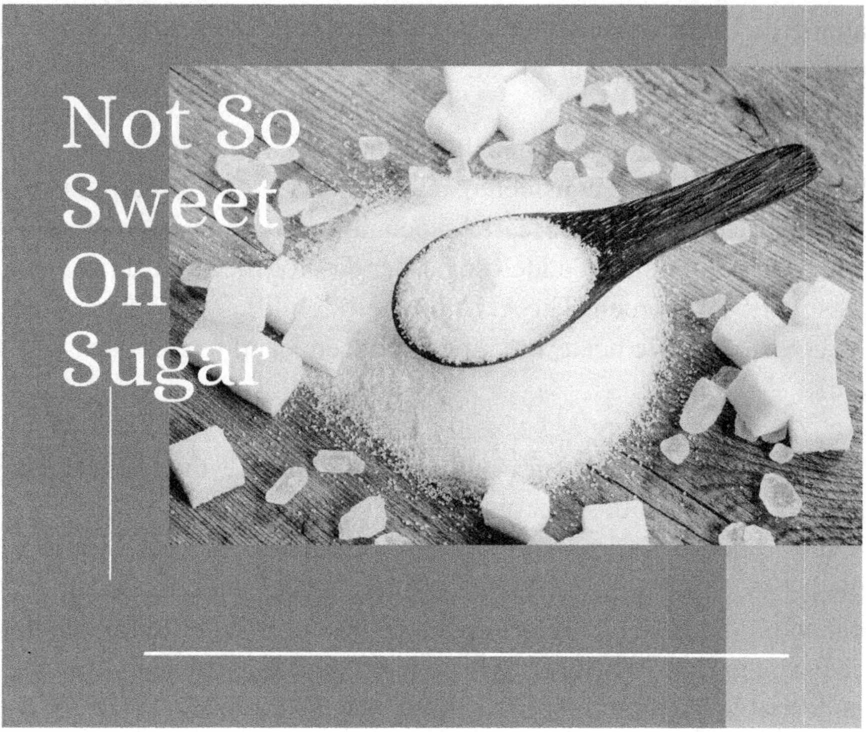

Chapter 5

The Not So Sweet on Sweets

We love our sugar! Unfortunately, we all pay the price because we love it so much. Modern diets are crammed with sugars and sweeteners. According to the American Heart Association, the average American consumes 22 teaspoons of added sugars daily in foods, drinks, and sweeteners. Varied reports indicate that Americans consume between 100 and 150 pounds of sugar annually. Unfortunately, this also includes children who eat three times their sugar weight a year.

No nutritional guidelines state how much sugar is needed daily because sugar is not considered an essential vitamin or nutrient. However, the American Heart Association recommends no more than nine teaspoons of added sugar per day for men and six teaspoons for women. The AHA limits for children vary depending on age and caloric needs but range between 3 and 6 teaspoons daily.

If we are talking about our health and microbiome, then we cannot neglect to talk about sugar and the damage it is causing to our bodies. The probiotics in our gut feed on prebiotics, which are plant-based fibers from whole foods like apples, onions, garlic, bananas, and oats. Can you guess what the harmful bacteria like to eat? You guessed it, sugar! When we eat a high-sugar diet, the undesirable bacteria thrive and grow out of control while our beneficial bacteria dwindle in numbers.

Not only are we dealing with the sugar epidemic, but we are also dealing with the sugar replacements epidemic. Sugar, whether it is an accurate sugar substitute or not, is considered a chemical that harms our bodies. Sugar substitutes are a neurotoxin and are killing our brains.

The problem with sugars, besides being so addictive, it raises havoc on our blood sugars. Sugar causes glucose to spike and drastically fall quickly. Sugar has been associated with heart problems, weight gain, insulin resistance, cancer, and severe inflammation.

Sugar can be considered toxic because it is an empty calorie. Sugar contains no vitamins or minerals. It has no extra nutrients to help the body processes it. During its processing, it sucks our bodies of vitamins and minerals, trying to flush it out.

Sugar is a carbohydrate, and our bodies need carbohydrates to survive. They are an essential form of energy. When we eat a carbohydrate, insulin from our pancreas is released to help move the sugar into our cells. The slower the process, the better. Whole grains do not break down into sugars quickly. White grains that have had the fiber removed break down into sugar quickly and react the same way to our bodies as to consuming regular sugar. When sugar is used quickly, it leaves extra insulin in the bloodstream for an extended time.

Although insulin is essential for our bodies, excess insulin causes increased inflammation and weight gain. This is one of the critical factors that lead to diabetes.

When discussing sugar, we often hear "Glucose and Fructose." So, what is the difference between them, and what is better for you?

Whenever our body takes any sugar, it must convert it into glucose. Glucose is the energy source for our bodies and is present in every cell. When we consume fructose, it must be converted into glucose for our bodies to use. The liver is the only organ that can metabolize fructose in significant amounts. Therefore, most fructose goes directly to the liver to be metabolized and turned into glucose. Because of this, too much fructose is very damaging to our liver. When the liver gets overloaded and unable to keep up with the demands of the conversion from fructose to glucose, it turns the fructose into extra fat. This is why fructose increases triglyceride levels.

So, if Fructose is so bad for you, why is fruit good? Yes, fruit is made with fructose, but it is only healthy for you when it is in its original form. A piece of fruit also contains fiber and other vitamins and enzymes. It is hard to consume too much fructose with fruit. Does this mean you can go crazy with the fruit? No! When counseling our patients and clients, we suggest around two servings of fruit a day.

There are many types of sugars in ingredients. It is essential to read all the labels. Below, we will list different kinds of sugars found in some products that you need to look out for and be aware of. This is where knowledge is so necessary. The more knowledge you have on this subject, the more you can decide what is best for your body.

Anhydrous dextrose
brown sugar
cane crystals
cane sugar
corn sweetener
corn syrup
corn syrup solids
crystal dextrose
evaporated cane juice
fructose sweetener
fruit juice concentrates
high-fructose corn syrup
honey
liquid fructose
malt syrup
maple syrup
molasses
pancake syrup
Rice Syrup
raw sugar
sugar
syrup
white sugar
fructose
lactose
Maltose

Remember that food companies have become very deceitful about what they put on labels. This list is not all-inclusive, and there are many more names that companies call added sugars.

Natural sweeteners

If you must use a sweetener, natural sources make the healthiest choices. You can adjust nearly any recipe to swap out regular table sugar for a more nutritious option. Honey, maple syrup, dates, coconut sugar, stevia, and fruit juice are some of the top choices for natural sweeteners.

Stevia

Stevia is a South American herb used as a sweetener by the Guarani Indians of Paraguay for hundreds of years. The leaves of the small, green Stevia plant has a delicious and refreshing taste that can be 30 times sweeter than sugar, but it has no calories and

Consuming it does not raise blood glucose levels or feed candida infections. Try using stevia as your primary source of sweetener in your foods and drinks.

Sugar Alcohols

Sugar alcohols occur naturally in plants. They are like sugar in some ways, but the body does not entirely absorb them. Because of this, they don't affect blood sugar levels as much and provide fewer calories per gram. Because they are not wholly absorbed, they can ferment in the intestines and cause extreme bloating, gas, or diarrhea.

Amino Acid Therapy

If your intense sugar cravings are due to low blood sugar, L-glutamine is an amino acid that can help. L-glutamine is a calming amino acid that can calm your cravings. It is best to take it in between meals. Start with a low dose and see how it works for you.

If you can find it in powder form when a craving arises, put a bit on your tongue, and your cravings will immediately disappear.

Many people say you need to avoid sugar completely, and some say you can have it in moderation. Do we think sugar will kill you? No! But what it does to your body over time can cause health problems much quicker. Because of this, be very wise with your sugar consumption. Look to see where you can eliminate and cut out sugar. Look to see where you can replace your item with natural sugars.

While working with our patients and clients, we have found that they crave sugar less when they replace all their sugar intake with natural sugars. They no longer need another sweet. One favorable thing for the consumer is that the foods also taste natural and are not processed.

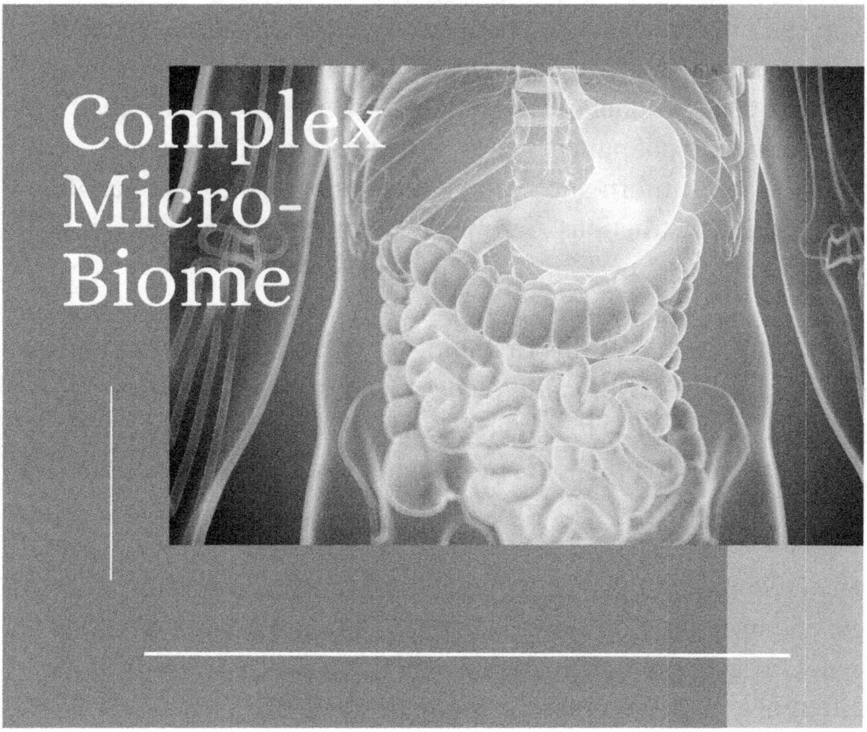

Chapter 6

Cutting Edge for the Microbiome

According to the National Human Genome Research Institute. The Human Genome Project (HGP) was an international, collaborative research program whose goal was the complete mapping and understanding of all the genes of human beings. All our genes together are known as our "Genome."

The HGP has revealed that there are about 20,500 human genes. The completed human sequence can now identify their locations. This ultimate product of the HGP has given the world detailed information about human genes' structure, organization, and function. This information can be thought of as the basic set of inheritable "Instructions" for the development and function of a human being.

A startling finding of this first draft was that the number of human genes appeared significantly fewer than previous estimates, ranging from 50,000 to as many as 140,000 genes.
This, along with long hours of listening to experts, was the beginning of microbiome research.

The HGP was astonished by how little we humans have in terms of genetic makeup. For example, rice, the plant, has over 40,000 genes. That is more than double a human's genes, yet look at the difference. It doesn't make sense until you look at the MicroBiome. Because of these critters, the human body has 100 times more gene expression that fulfills many of our essential needs.

Genetic testing has also improved significantly in the last decade. Science and technology have drastically increased, and we can now have genetic testing for only a few hundred dollars. The technology for testing gut microbes has advanced as well. Although more needs to be done on these tests, we now have science that can show what our MicroBiome is doing and what creatures are affecting our health.

In an often-cited Harvard study published in 2010, researchers examined the effect of diet on the microbiome by evaluating the gut bacteria of children in rural Africa. These children eat a higher-fiber diet similar to that of early human settlements. The scientists used genetic tests to identify the types of bacteria in the children's feces. In addition, they found short-chain fatty acids, which are manufactured by gut bacteria when they digest plant fiber called polysaccharides.

The two largest groups of bacteria are Firmicutes and Bacteroidetes. Together, they make up 90% of the gut population. The ratio of these two groups determines inflammation levels and relates to conditions such as obesity, heart disease, and inflammation in general. The higher ratio of Firmicutes to Bacteroidetes is strongly associated with more inflammation and obesity.

Firmicutes bacteria are exceptionally adept at extracting calories from food to increase caloric absorption. Weight gain is more likely if your body can absorb more calories from your food as it moves through the gastrointestinal tract. Bacteroidetes, on the other hand, specialize in breaking down plant starches and fibers into short fatty acid molecules that the body can use for energy. The Harvard study showed that the Western guts had more Firmicutes, thus leading to much more obesity in our population.

Dr. David Perlmutter, MD, published These studies in the book Brain Maker.

Now, to go even a little more in-depth, we have all heard of a heart transplant. Liz's father had a heart transplant at age 65. There are other organs like the liver, kidney, lung, and so forth that can be transplanted. Usually, this occurs when one has passed away, and the organ is transplanted into one who is in desperate need of help.

There is another transplant on the rise that could directly change the makeup of the microbiome: Fecal Microbial Transplant, FMT for short. That is correct, transplanting POOP. In the United States, at this time, it can only be done for severe cases of C-diff. However, it is being done in Europe and other areas to address many health problems, and it has had remarkable results. FMT

It is precisely what it is: transferring a healthy person's fecal matter with good microbiota into an unhealthy, sometimes severely sick person's digestive tract to help repopulate their gut with better bacteria. This leads to much better health. It sounds gross or extreme, but this procedure has drastically changed people's lives.

I have a good friend from Chiropractic School who had a devastating reaction to the antibiotic Cipro. The last 16 months have been pure hell because of the toxicity that occurred with this medication. It destroyed his MicroBiome. His health and brain function have been in severe decline. So, at this time, it has only been one week post-FMT, and he is already noticing more significant changes than anything he has previously tried.

Over the next several years, this practice will become much more widely known and may even become standard procedure. Most, if not all, diseases and sickness start in the gut because of reduced function of the microbiome. If we directly focus on the microbiome and get to the underlying cause, I believe, like many others, that we will see significant advancements in our health care.

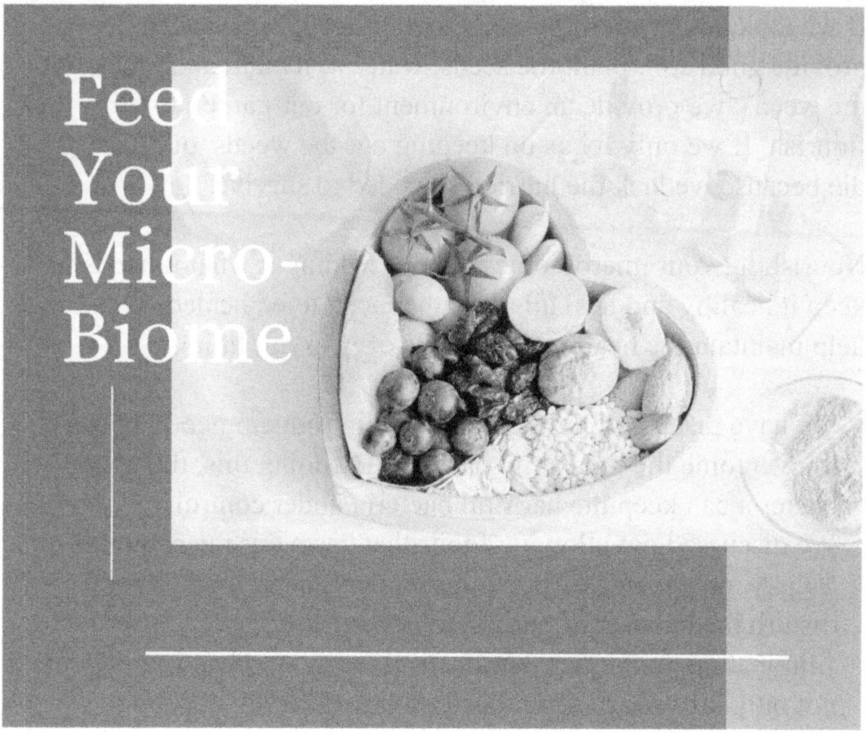

Chapter Seven

Nourishing the MicroBiome - Gut

Nourishing your microbiome is just as important as removing the toxic ingredients. It creates an environment for your microbiome to flourish, helps eliminate leaky gut, keeps the good guys vibrant and alive, and maintains a healthy balance between good and bad bugs.

If we look at our microbiome, we often see it as a garden. If we provide good soil, plant the seeds, water it, feed it, and pluck out the weeds, we provide an environment for our garden to grow and flourish. If we only focus on keeping out the weeds, our garden can die because we lack the nutrients needed to survive.

Nourishing your microbiome is about feeding it what it needs to keep it healthy and heal all areas that need to be healed. This can help maintain the health of the walls of your gut lining.

- We have discussed fermentation and introducing good bacteria to overcome the unhealthy bacteria. By doing this, the good bacteria can keep the harmful bacteria under control.
- We discussed not allowing foods that harm our microbiome. Sugary, processed, GMO, and chemical-laden foods can all disturb the balance of our microbiome.
- Eliminating antibiotics, antibacterial soap, and hand sanitizers all not only kills the harmful bacteria but also kills the good bacteria.
- We have also discussed the critical role of sound and proper probiotics.

Now that we have established a healthy environment, how do we continue to nourish it? There are many ways to do this, but we have found two very helpful.

Aloe Vera

Aloe vera has been used for centuries to aid healing. It can easily be considered a superfood, rich in vitamins, minerals, amino acids, enzymes, and antioxidants.

Just like it heals cuts on your skin, it also heals cuts on your stomach lining. It nourishes the walls to create healthy, thick walls.

Aloe vera reduces inflammation by soothing and relaxing the GI tract. It also relieves constipation and promotes regular bowel movements. Aloe vera also has antibacterial and antiviral properties.

Aloe Vera should be used consistently to help nourish your gut lining. We use aloe Vera almost every day. It is very versatile and easy to add to any drink. You can purchase a live plant, liquid drinks, or in a pill form.

Using a live plant is easier than it sounds. Cut off a stem, remove the gel, and put it in water. Aloe vera can also be purchased in 100% juice. You can either drink this juice straight or add it to any drink. If you are purchasing gel, do not get the gel that has other additives added to it. These contain chemicals that can be harmful to your body.

We started using liquid aloe vera several years ago when Dr. Watt heard about it helping with allergies in an infomercial. This was way before he knew anything about gut health. It was a natural way to help, so he tried it. Several months before allergy season, he started drinking straight aloe vera juice. Sure enough, he has been allergy-free ever since.

Bone Broth

Bone Broth is a mineral-rich infusion made by boiling the bones of healthy animals with vegetables, herbs, and spices. Many are skeptical when they hear bone broth, but it has existed for many years. Remember how you would eat chicken soup when you were sick? The tradition continued, but the way it was prepared needed to be recovered. Many societies worldwide still consume bone broth regularly as it is a cheap and highly nutrient-dense food.

Bone broth can help improve digestion, allergies, immune health, brain health, and more. Many consider homemade, nutrient-dense bone broth a superfood. Not only is it a superfood, but it is also straightforward and inexpensive to make.

There is no comparison to the store-bought versions. Most store-bought broths contain MSG or other chemicals, and many lack gelatin and other important health-boosting properties of homemade broth.

Bone Broth supplies the broken-down materials from cartilage and tendons, such as glucosamine and chondroitin, which assist the joints in the body. Consuming bone broth supplies natural gelatin to the diet. Because of this, cartilage, bone and joints, skin, digestive tract, and muscles, including the heart, benefit.

In addition to all the bone broth nutrition described above, one of the most beneficial products of bone broth is its ability to help the body with its detoxification. This is due to the large amounts of amino acids. Some of the many amino acids in bone broth consist of glycine, arginine, glutamine, and proline. Glycine is essential because it assists the liver in clearing out unnecessary toxins.

Our liver has to process and expel most of the toxins in our body. It is highly overworked. Given the toxicity of our world today and the elevated level of chemicals in our air, water, and food, our liver must be detoxing regularly. Glycine plays a significant role in detoxifying the liver so that we can maintain our health. Minerals are also in abundance. These minerals act as a chelator.

Different animal bones have specific properties and nutrients for your individual needs. For example, beef bone broth will help your joints, while chicken bone broth is more healing on the stomach. Fish bones help to focus on restoring the collagen in the skin.

Choose which area you want to work on and use those bones to produce the desired results.

In selecting the bones for bone broth, look for high-quality bones from grass-fed cattle or bison, pastured poultry, or wild-caught fish. Since you'll be extracting and drinking the minerals in concentrated form, you want to ensure the animal is as healthy as possible. Quality is essential to avoid issues with toxins and heavy metals. The way we look at it and teach it to our patients and clients is that the closer that animal is to its natural habitat, the better the bones will be.

The Process of Making Bone Broth

Remove all skins from bones unless you are using an organic carcass. Some skin can house toxins, so it is best to remove it. Meat can be left on the bone, but it is not necessary.

Place bones in a large stock or crock pot and cover with filtered water. Before cooking, add two tablespoons of raw apple cider vinegar or one lemon to the water. This raises the broth's acidic level, helping break down the bones and pull out the important nutrients inside them.

Add vegetables, herbs, and spices for added nutrition and flavor. Some suggestions to add to your broth are carrots, celery, onion, garlic, parsley, cilantro, bay leaf, basil, lemongrass, mineral salt, and peppercorns. My favorite foods are onion, garlic, cilantro, lemongrass, and mineral salt. Be creative and add what your taste buds love.

Bring to a boil, then reduce heat to a simmer. Each type of bone requires a specific simmering time to extract its nutrients fully. Follow these guidelines to determine the appropriate simmering duration for different types of bones:

- Fish bones, being thin and fragile, should simmer for about 12 hours.

- Chicken bones require around 24 hours.

- Beef bones, being dense and thick, should simmer for approximately 48 hours.

  Use these guidelines to determine the simmering time for the bones you use.

After the time is complete, strain the broth with a strainer. Discard the vegetables. The bones can either be discarded or returned to the freezer and reused. We recommend using your bones at most twice. If your broth is not gelatinous, discard your bones and use new ones for your next batch.

Just a side note: If you choose to use the vegetables and not discard them, cook your bone broth for your allotted time without them. After the broth is complete, strain your bones. Pour your clear bone broth back into your crockpot and add vegetables. Simmer on low until the vegetables become soft. Your broth will not be as flavorful cooking the entire time without the vegetables, but you will still get nutrients if you eat the vegetables with your broth.

Bone broth is very versatile. It can be used anywhere water is available; many people see the benefits.

I like sipping bone broth in a mug. Cooking with it is very easy and adds flavor to your dishes. You can incorporate bone broth into your cooking, including soups and sauces.

Both aloe vera and bone broth create a healing, nourishing environment to heal your gut and stay healthy. They help keep your system strong to withstand any invaders. Your garden cannot grow unless you nourish it and strengthen it.

Aloe vera and bone broth heal and help fix damaged gut and intestinal tract walls. By implementing these strategies, your microbiome and gut can be strong enough to withstand the wind that comes its way.

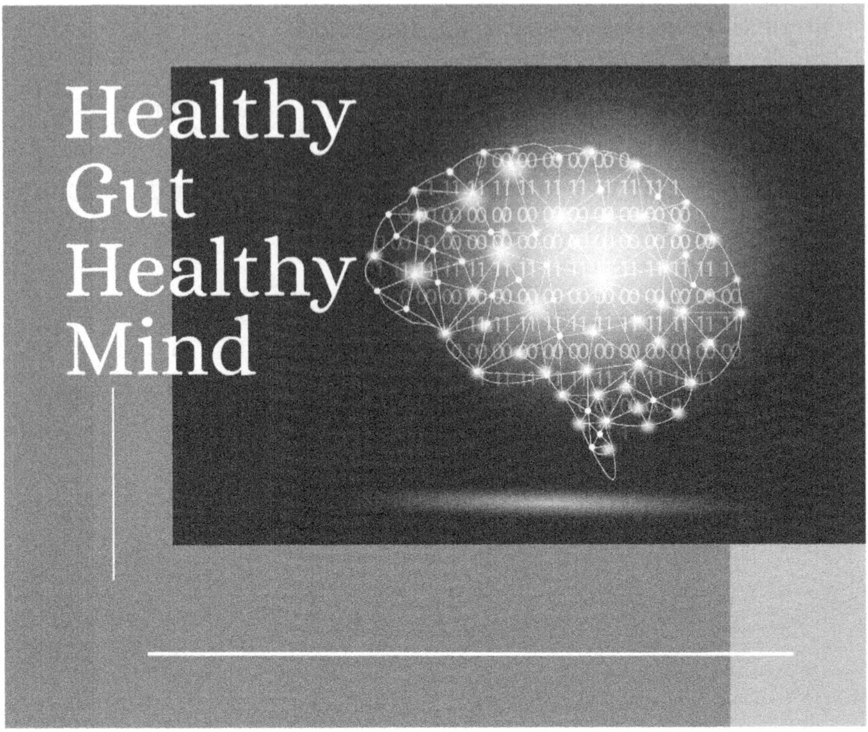

Chapter Eight

Healthy Mind

The microbiome is known as the second brain. What is going on in your gut is also in your mind. When your mind is not functioning correctly, we know your brain is unhealthy. Many people who suffer from anxiety and depression also suffer from a gut problem. Often, Dr. Watt helps his patients heal their gut, and their anxiety and depression drastically decrease and even go away.

While the second brain doesn't get involved in actual thought processes, it does control behavior on its own. Researchers believe this is because it allows our bodies to make digestion more efficient. Instead of sending digestion responses through the spinal cord to the brain and back, we developed a brain within our gut that could handle things closer to the source.

One thing we know for sure is that our gut is directly affected by our brain. Our thoughts and emotions send signals to our gut. Stress, for example, is intimately tied to our gut via the vagus nerve. Our bodies respond to stress with a "fight or flight" system.

When something scary happens, or you begin to worry, you react physically. Have you ever seen police lights in your rearview mirror, and suddenly, your stomach gets sick, your palms get sweaty, and your heartbeat starts to race? A shot of adrenaline Cortisol is released into the system from the adrenal glands. Generally, nausea comes from the release of epinephrine, more commonly known as "adrenaline." This disrupts the stomach and intestines' acids, enzymes, and functions. Your thoughts and emotions are directly tied to your gut.

If you're in a stressful situation, your body reacts, you deal with the problem, and then your body returns to normal. Unfortunately, if you're constantly stressed, your body is stuck in the fight or flight phase over an extended period.

Our bodies are unable to distinguish between physical and mental stress. They would respond the same way if a bear appeared in our home as when we were stressed about our jobs. Our bodies will always act the same way to combat stress.

This constant state of stress, combined with unbalanced hormone regulation, causes chronic inflammation. When stressed, your body constantly tries to fix the problem, like a festering wound. Stress can lead to inflammation, and inflammation is known as the root of many diseases.

Prolonged exposure to stress can have severe consequences for your health. These symptoms can range from high blood pressure to autoimmune disorders. The microbiome is directly affected by the inflammation within our gut. Because of this, our microbiome is directly affected by our immune response. Improvement of the gut can drastically improve your mental well-being.

What Are Ways We Can Improve Our Gut-Brain Connection?

1- Diet: Focus on getting all vitamins and minerals from natural food sources

2- Eat Probiotics: Get your probiotics through your fermented foods or over-the-counter probiotics

3- Avoid gluten: Most people have an inflammatory response to gluten. If you are one of them or you don't know if you are, stay away from gluten and evaluate your body, gut, and mind connection

4- Eat healthy fats: Fats are food for your brain. They help stabilize your metabolism and don't increase your blood sugar, which can damage your brain.

5- B6 vitamins: Vitamin B6 impacts the production of serotonin and neurotransmitters. Healthy B6 levels are associated with a positive mood and naturally reduce stress.

6- Nuts: Nuts are full of serotonin, the happy-feeling chemicals in your brain. They are an excellent snack for a combination of proteins and fats.

7- Amino Acids: Each neurotransmitter has its pathway and uses different amino acids. Three of the major pathways are the serotonin pathway, the dopamine/ norepinephrine pathway, and the GABA pathway. Amino Acids, such as Tyrosine, Tryptophan, and many others, are essential protein building blocks for the brain.

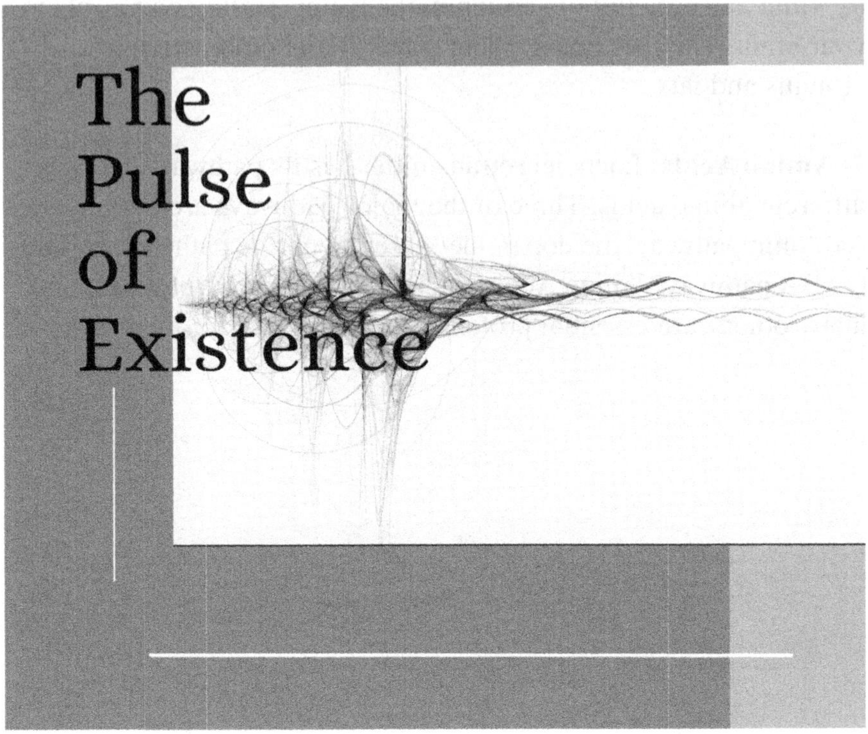

Chapter Nine

Different Foods Different Vibrations

We have to end this book by explaining how it started. Nutrition is a critical component of our overall health. No supplement can replace the nutrition you get from your foods. Our bodies are designed to get nutrients from their natural sources. Yes, some things are out of our control; this is where supplementation comes into play. But our first defense should be the foods we eat. This is where your healing will occur.

Every food we eat has a vibrational frequency that communicates with our bodies on a cellular level. There are high-vibrational foods and low-vibrational foods. Our health is directly correlated to these vibrational foods we eat.

Recent studies have demonstrated how different foods change the body's energy field. It is no coincidence that the best foods for you increase that energy field, and the foods that are not good for you decrease it. Studying this energy, known as "Quantum Physics," will be a crucial part of understanding our health in the future.

Part of taking responsibility for our health is evaluating these foods and noticing their vibration level in our bodies. Through this process, we become more aware of how each food affects us and our health.

Because everyone has a different energetic makeup, various foods can bring different vibrations to other people. Only you truly know what will make you feel good in your skin and create a positive vibration. The best part is that you are in control and get to be the judge. So, tune in!

When starting this process, it is easy to start with a list of documented higher-vibrational foods and work from there. High-vibrational foods are typically in their purest, most natural form and are connected to the earth. An organic apple directly off the tree will have a higher vibration than the ones already cut up in a bag with some preservatives at your local grocery store.

Below is a list of high-vibrational foods that have been tested. Notice how each is associated with the earth. All of them have yet to be processed.

- Fresh organic fruits and vegetables
- Dark leafy greens
- Fresh-pressed green juice
- Pure clean water
- Raw nuts & seeds
- Coconut
- Free range eggs
- Wild fish
- Raw oils like extra virgin olive oil, coconut oil
- Sea vegetation
- Raw honey
- Maple syrup
- Fermented foods
- Sprouted foods
- Spirulina (Green powders)
- Herbs & Spices
- Herbal teas
- Legumes
- Grains such as buckwheat, brown rice, amaranth, Quinoa

This is only a short list but a great place to start. Your quest is to find what foods work best for you and your body. We have had many patients and clients who could not tolerate even some of these foods. This is why you must evaluate your body and each individual's vibration level.

How do you find the vibrational level of the foods you eat? This is where your homework comes into play. You can't always rely on someone to tell you what is good or bad for you. You are the only one who knows. Because of this, you must put in the work and write up your list.

Take a journal and write out a food log. At the top of a page, put down the food you will be testing for your body. It is essential to be honest with yourself through this process. The more honest you are, the better this exercise will work.

Let's say you are going to test for an apple. Begin by writing "Apple" at the top of your page. Below this, specify the apple you are testing, for example, "Red Delicious." It's important to note the variety because different types of apples can have varying effects on your body. For instance, I have noticed that my body reacts more sensitively to Granny Smith apples than Gala apples. This initial identification helps in understanding how specific varieties influence your physical responses.

Step 1: Hold an apple and observe your body's reaction. Tune into the sensations and messages your body communicates to you. Notice any feelings or responses that arise. While this might sound unconventional, it's based on the idea that your body has a memory associated with each food you've encountered. By holding the apple, your body may naturally recall and react based on past experiences with this fruit.

In your journal, write down what you felt and how your body reacted to the apple. Then, give this food a number from 1 to 10 (10 being the highest).

Step 2: As you eat the apple, engage fully with the experience. Pay close attention to how it affects your body. Notice whether you feel an increase in energy or if it seems to diminish. What sensations or messages is the apple conveying to your body? Record your observations in your journal as you eat, noting any physical or emotional responses.

Alongside your notes, rate your experience on a scale from 1 to 10. This mindfulness practice will help you attune to your body's unique reactions to different foods.

Step 3: 30-Minute Check-In
30 minutes after consumption, assess your feelings. Note any changes in your energy levels or physical sensations. Record these observations in your journal and assign a rating from 1 to 10, with 1 being minimal impact and 10 being significant.

Step 4: 60-Minute Evaluation
An hour after eating the apple, reflect on your physical and emotional state again. Are there any new sensations or continued effects from the apple? Document your findings in your journal, providing a similar rating based on the intensity of your reactions.

Step 5: 2-Hour Assessment
Two hours post-consumption, perform a final evaluation of your body's response to the apple. This longer interval can help capture delayed reactions or subtle changes that may not have been apparent earlier. Write down your observations and complete your entries with a corresponding number from 1 to 10.

These steps will help you gauge your body's responses over time, offering valuable insights into how foods like apples influence your well-being beyond the immediate eating experience.

Once you have completed your food journal, each food item will have a series of numbers associated with its effects at different stages. To determine the overall "vibration level" of each food for your body, sum these numbers. Then, multiply the total by 2. This will give you a vibration level score between 1 and 100.

For example, if your total for a specific food is 32, multiply that by 2 to reach a vibration level of 64 out of 100. Based on this method, our target is to consume foods with a vibration level of at least 80. A score of 64 indicates that the food may not be optimal for you, suggesting a need to find a healthier substitute that better aligns with your body's needs.

The more you practice this process, the better you will become at it. Practice makes perfect. By the end of this exercise, you will understand what foods sit well with your body and which items you should substitute for better options. As you continue this practice, you will become more in tune with your body and its needs for a healthy life.

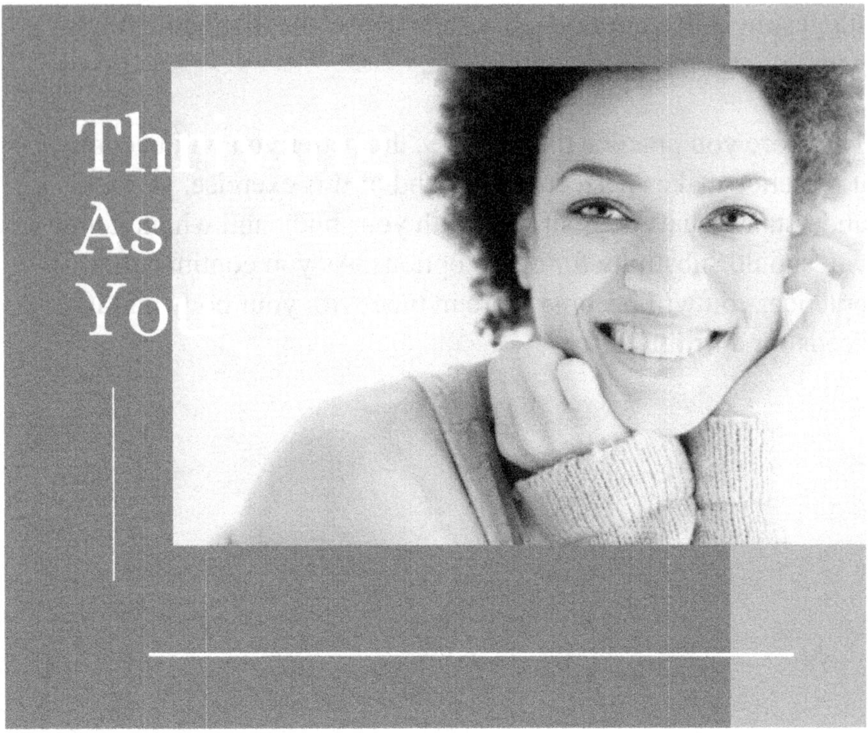

Chapter Ten

Being Your Best Self

Health is what we put in our bodies and how we treat and care for them. Being healthy requires a perfect connection with our mind, body, and soul. Our connection to ourselves will increase as we practice mindful eating, learn new ideas, and educate ourselves about our minds and bodies.

As we become more attuned to our inner selves, we perceive a presence more significant than ourselves. We embrace the profound belief that our existence on this earth is for a sacred purpose. This connection to our inner self and something transcendent allows us to operate from a place of love and respect for ourselves and those around us.

Self-respect teaches us that our actions are significant and that we play a crucial role in the tapestry of life. This understanding makes us more inclined to make choices that nurture our minds, bodies, and spirits. We select foods that fuel us, engage in activities that enrich us, and foster relationships that support our growth. This holistic approach enhances our well-being and aligns us with our fundamental mission on earth.

Healing begins within, a fundamental principle we must cherish. We are bestowed with the incredible gift of life. Our bodies are marvels of nature; each cell is intricately designed to support who we are.

Intrinsically, our bodies possess the wisdom to heal, provided they are in the right environment. Ultimately, the responsibility to nurture and love our bodies falls upon us. It is our duty to care for them comprehensively, ensuring we create conditions where our bodies not only survive but are thriving.

We hope this book has provided valuable knowledge and insights to honor your health and body. By implementing what you've learned, even minor adjustments can lead to significant improvements. Remember, life is not merely to be lived; it is to be fully experienced. We each have only one body, yet it holds immense potential to drive positive change in the world. Seize this opportunity to live the life you were meant to lead and to become the person you were destined to be. When we are at our healthiest, we gain the sacred privilege to assist and uplift others.

Dr. Shane and Liz Watt

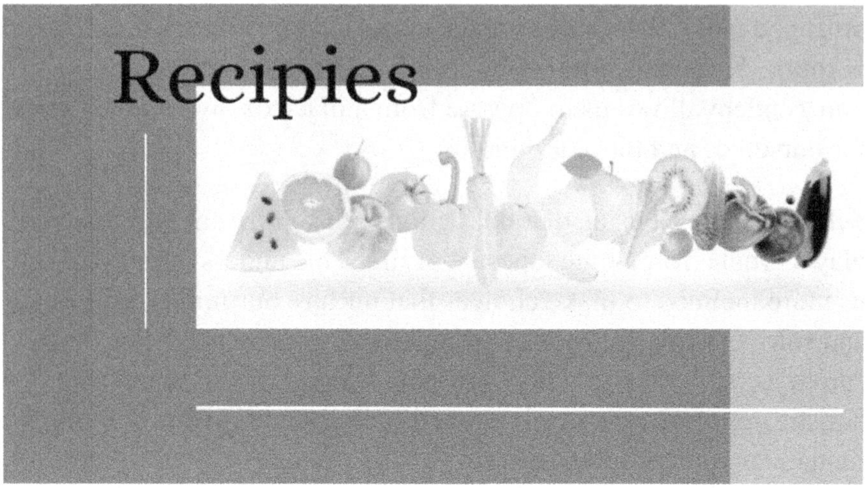

Recipes

Vegetable Fermentation

Summer Salad

2 Heads of Green Cabbage
1 Large Carrot
1 Red Bell Pepper
1 Bunch Cilantro
1/2 Bunch Italian Parsley
2 Stalks Celery
2-3 Tbsp Real or Himalayan Salt

Prepare the Vegetables:

- Shred the cabbage, carrot, and pepper. Place them in a large glass bowl.
- Finely chop the cilantro and Italian parsley and add them to the shredded vegetables.

Make the Brine:

- Juice the celery to produce celery juice.
- Dissolve salt in the celery juice by stirring thoroughly.

Combine and Sit:

- Pour the celery juice mixture over the vegetables in the bowl. Stir the mixture until all vegetables are well coated.
- Allow the mixture to sit for 20-30 minutes. During this time, the vegetables will release water, creating additional brine.

Jar and Submerge:

- Transfer the vegetable mixture to a glass canning jar. Use a tamper or the back of a spoon to press down the vegetables, ensuring they are compacted and fully submerged in the brine.
- Release any trapped air bubbles by running a butter knife around the inside edge of the jar.
- Place whole cabbage leaves over the vegetables to help keep them submerged. If needed, add carrot stumps on top of these leaves.
- Ensure all vegetables are completely submerged in the liquid before tightly sealing the jar with a lid.

Fermentation:

- Place the sealed jar in a deep dish pan to catch any overflow. Leave it on your counter for 5-7 days. Check periodically for the desired level of crunchiness.

Hot Carrots

5-8 large carrots
large onion
2 jalapeno peppers
1/4 tsp. red pepper flakes
1 Tbsp salt
2 cups water

Prepare the Vegetables:

- Thinly slice carrots, onion, and jalapeño.
- Place the sliced vegetables into a clean glass quart jar.

Make the Brine:

- In a separate bowl, dissolve salt in water to create a brine solution.

Combine and Submerge:

- Pour the brine over the vegetables in the jar, ensuring they are covered. If necessary, top off with extra water to completely cover the vegetables.
- Add red pepper flakes to the jar and stir gently to distribute.

Ensure Submersion:

- Place a whole cabbage leaf or a large slice of onion on top of the vegetables to submerge them under the brine.
- Add carrot stumps or onion on top of the leaf to help weigh down the vegetables.

Ferment:

- Seal the jar tightly with a lid.
- Set the jar in a deep dish on your counter to catch any overflow, and allow the vegetables to ferment for five days.

Storage:

- After five days, check the vegetables for desired taste and crunchiness. Once ready, store the jar in the refrigerator.

Dressings

Healthy Vinaigrette

3/4 cup olive oil
1 cup red wine or strawberry vinegar
2 tsp garlic powder
2 tsp oregano
2 tsp basil
1 1/2 tsp pepper
1 1/2 tsp Himalayan salt
1 1/2 tsp onion powder
1 1/2 tsp Dijon mustard
Combine all ingredients in a blender until smooth

Cilantro Lime Dressing

One head of fresh cilantro
1/8 cup dried chopped onions
1 cup avocado oil
2 Tbsp raw apple cider vinegar
1/4 tsp natural stevia powder
1/2 tsp true lime
1/2 tsp Himalayan salt
Put all ingredients in a blender and blend until smooth

Sweet Poppy Seed Dressing

1 cup avocado oil
1/3 cup raw apple cider vinegar
1/4 cup dried onions
1/4 tsp real stevia
1/2 tsp Himalayan salt
1 Tablespoons poppy seeds
Put all ingredients in a blender and blend

Creamy Cilantro Dressing

1 cup homemade mayonnaise
1 cup kefir
One head cilantro
¼ tsp dried dill
¼ c dried onion
1 tsp Himalayan salt
¼ tsp pepper
Pinch paprika
Put all ingredients in a blender and blend
Soups

Soups

Basic Cream Sauce

1 cup raw cashews
3 cups water
1 tsp tapioca flour
1/2 salt

Cream of Chicken- Add 1 Tbsp Better than Bullion chicken stock and shredded chicken

Creamy Parmesan- Add 1/2 c parmesan cheese and 1/2 tsp dried basil

Sweet Cream- Add 2 Tbsp of sweetener of choice

Curry- Add 1 Tbsp Curry powder and 1/2 tsp turmeric, 1 Tbsp Better Than Bullion chicken broth

Put on medium heat on the stove. Stir on low boil until thick.

Italian Potato Soup

6 cups water
2 Tbsp. Better Than Bullion
6 oz. ground natural sausage
One onion
Four large potatoes
½ tsp red pepper flakes
3 cups chopped kale
I batch basic cream sauce
Salt (Himalayan) and pepper to taste

Brown sausage and onion in a soup pot. Add the rest of the ingredients except cream sauce and kale. When potatoes are tender, add cream sauce and kale. Salt and pepper to taste.

Chicken Curry Soup

2 cups shredded cooked chicken
6 cups water
2 Tbsp Better Than Bullion
One leek sliced
½ red pepper chopped
One medium onion chopped
½ cup coconut flakes
One can of green chilies
1 Tbsp curry
¼ tsp turmeric
1 tsp Himalayan salt
One coarsely chopped tomato
1 batch of basic cream sauce
One whole head of cilantro chopped
One fresh lime squeezed
1 Tbsp honey

Add water, chicken, Better Than Bullion, Leak, red pepper, onion, coconut flakes, green chilies, curry, turmeric, and salt in a soup pot. Boil on medium until vegetables are tender. When tender, add the rest of the ingredients.

Tuscan White Bean Soup

1 Tbsp olive oil
One onion
Three cloves garlic
6 cups water
2 tsp dried basil
1 tsp sage
1 cup coarsely chopped sun-dried tomatoes
3 cups cooked white beans
2 Tbsp Better Than Bullion
½ tsp red pepper flakes
A batch of basil cream sauce

3 cups combination of kale and spinach and fresh basil
In a stock pot, sauté oil with onion and garlic. Add the rest of the ingredients and simmer until well combined. Salt to taste.

Breads

Bean tortillas

1 cup Bob's Red Mill All Purpose Bean Flour
1 cup water
2 Tbsp nutritional yeast
1/2 tsp salt
1/4 tsp dried turmeric
1/2 tsp garlic blend seasoning

Mix ingredients. In an 8-inch saucepan over medium heat, put 1/3 c of the mixture in the pan and swish around, forming a thin circle. When the edges begin to lift, turn over.

Pizza Crust

1 cup oats
1 cup gluten-free ancient grain flour
Two eggs
1 tsp sea salt
1 tsp dried basil
1 tsp fresh garlic
1 cup water

Mix ingredients. The mixture will be sticky. Shape into a circle with a fork on stone or parchment paper. Bake at 350 for 15 minutes or until golden brown. Top with your favorite toppings!

Oatmeal Pumpkin Pancakes

One ripe banana
Three eggs
1/4 cup Coconut oil
1/4 tsp Salt

1 tsp Vanilla
1 Tbsp Pumpkin spice

Mix well in blender. Add 1 cup of oats. After well-blended, add 1/2 teaspoon baking powder. Cook on a medium skillet.

Dishes

Butternut Squash Dish

2 cups soaked brown rice
One can of coconut milk
2 cups steamed butternut squash
2 cups cooked, sprouted black beans
One avocado diced
One head of chopped cilantro
1/2 cup feta cheese
1 tsp Mexican salt

Soak the rice for 4 hours, drain it, and add coconut milk and one can of water. On low, cook the rice for about 45 minutes until cooked all through. Add the rest of the ingredients to a big salad bowl and enjoy.

Quinoa Mexican Dish

2 cups quinoa cooked
1 cup meat (sausage, hamburger, chicken)
One onion
1/2 cup red and yellow peppers
One can of green chilies
1 Tbsp cumin
1/2 tsp chili powder
2 cups salsa

Sauté onion and peppers with meat. Add the rest of the ingredients. Stir well and put in a large pie pan. Cover with Salsa. You can sprinkle it with cheese and a dollop of sour cream or Kefir cheese as an extra.

Chicken Curry and Vegetables over Rice

Prepared curry sauce (recipe above)
Chopped vegetables such as potatoes, peppers, squash, onions, and peas
prepared Rice
Add vegetables and shredded chicken to the prepared curry sauce. Pour over rice.

Cilantro Lime sprouted lentils

1 Tbsp avocado oil or coconut oil
2 cups sprouted green lentils
1/4 tsp True Lime Seasoning
2 tsp dried cilantro

In a saucepan with oil, sauté all ingredients for 5 minutes. It can be a side dish or a substitute for rice.

Healthy Cafe Rio Pork

One large pork roast
3 cups of tomatoes
2 inches fresh pineapple
One medium onion
One head cilantro
2 Tbsp molasses
1 tsp sea salt
2 tsp chili powder
2 Tbsp cumin

Put a pot roast in a pressure cooker. In a Vitamix or blender, puree the rest of the ingredients until smooth. Pour over the top of the roast and bring to pressure. Cook for 1 hour. When finished, shred the pork. If you want a slow cooker, cook for 6 to 8 hours on High.

Homemade Enchilada sauce

1 Tbsp Avocado Oil
Four cloves of garlic
One onion divided
Two large tomatoes
1/8 tsp cayenne powder
2 tsp oregano
2 tsp cumin
Three tomatoes
3/4 cup water or bone broth

Sauté 1 Tablespoon Avocado Oil with four cloves of garlic. Blend the garlic mixture and the rest of the ingredients in a blender. Simmer the mixture in a pan for 15 to 30 minutes.

Enchiladas

Enchilada sauce
Bean tortillas
Grilled diced Chicken
One head of Cilantro chopped
One cup of cooked sprouted black beans
1/2 cup shredded Extra Sharp Cheddar cheese
1/4 cup Feta Cheese
1/2 head of lettuce chopped.

Preheat the oven to 350*. Combine the grilled chicken, chopped cilantro, and black beans. Place the mixture in bean tortillas and place them in a pan. Pour the sauce over the top, sprinkle with extra sharp cheddar cheese, and sprinkle with Feta cheese. Bake until the cheese is melted. Serve over chopped lettuce.

Desserts

Oatmeal Banana Chocolate Chip Cookies

3 cups oats
Two eggs
Two very ripe bananas
1/4 cup molasses
1/2 tsp baking soda
1/2 tsp salt
1/2 cup coconut oil
1/2 cup chopped pecans
1 cup chocolate chips

Preheat oven to 325*. Mix all ingredients in Vitamix until well blended. Add chocolate chips and nuts.
With a cookie scoop, place on parchment paper. Bake for 15 min. Place on a cooling rack.

Protein balls

1 cup peanut butter
1/2 cup honey
1/2 cup oats blended
four scoops of chocolate protein powder
1/2 unsweetened coconut flakes

Combine all ingredients. Roll it into a ball and put it into the fridge.

Chocolate Coconut Bombs
1/2 cup coconut oil
1/4 cup organic cocoa
1/4 cup unsweetened coconut flakes
1/4 tsp natural stevia powder
1/4 tsp maple syrup (optional)
1/4 tsp almond extract (optional)
Chopped pecans
Unsweetened Coconut Flakes

Combine coconut oil, cocoa, unsweetened coconut flakes, stevia powder, maple syrup, and almond extract. Roll into balls and coat with pecans and coconut flakes; refrigerate.

Food Journaling

Food

Food

Food

Food

Food

Food

Food

Food

Food

Food

Food

Food

Food

Food

Food

Food____

____

____

____

Food____

____

____

____

Food____

____

____

____

Food____

____

____

____

Food____

____

____

____

____

Food

Food

Food

Food

Food

Food

Food

Food

Food

Food

Self Reflection

How has my perspective on health and wellness changed?

What first steps can I take to implement what I've learned?

Which dietary changes am I most excited to try?

What obstacles might I face, and how can I overcome them?

How will I track my progress on this journey?

Who can support me in making these changes?

What has been the most surprising information I've discovered?

How can I integrate these practices into my daily routine?

What long-term goals do I have for my health?

How can I involve my family in this journey toward better health?

Contact The Authors

Dr. M Shane Watt
Mountain West Chiropractic
Neurobolic Health Center
1664 West Town Center Drive
South Jordan, Utah 84095
drmswatt@yahoo.com
www.watthealth.com
801-446-0800

Liz Watt
ElizabethAnnWatt.com
Liz@ElizabethAnnWatt.com
@LizWattSpeaks
801-755-2457

Be Healthy Utah
BeHealthyUtah.com
@Be.Healthy.Utah
@BeHealthyUSA

Made in the USA
Monee, IL
04 November 2026

67377419R00049